How To Spot The Gout Danger Zone

Graham Alexander

Copyright © 2015 Jayu Worldwide Ltd

All rights reserved.

ISBN: 1508843074
ISBN-13: 978-1508843078

To my wonderful little lady who grows
prettier every day.

CONTENTS

	An Early Warning System For Gout?	i
1	What is Gout?	1
2	Taking Pills	6
3	Alcohol	8
4	Diet	12
5	Cooking Style	19
6	Fasting	22
7	Hydration	24
8	Heat	26
9	The Gout Danger Zone Checklist	31
10	The Emergency Cupboard	36
11	Effective Action	40

AN EARLY WARNING SYSTEM FOR GOUT?

Feeling like your foot or toe is going to explode in pain is perhaps one of the most difficult things to express in words. It is a pain like no other that can reduce the strongest of men to tears. It makes us all beg and plead for an end to the invisible torment. Years ago I was laid up off work with my ankle in agony thinking how does this happen?

How does a condition so life changing happen without warning?

Wouldn't it be marvellous if I could spot gout before it happened?

This is when I started to take note. I kept watch on what my body was going through before each attack and slowly started to build a clear picture of how gout silently, painlessly appears before it attacks.

Through much research and trial and error, and excruciating pain, many sleepless nights and days off work I began to formulate a full understanding of the secret signs of gout.

1 WHAT IS GOUT?

Answer: Simply put gout is an acid problem.

Now I am not a doctor, scientist or researcher so the language that I use here to describe what is happening may not be to the liking of the medical profession. The aim here is to speak to you, the gout sufferer and make it easy for you to understand what is happening, not to impress medical professionals ☺.

Unlike most doctors and health specialists who only have textbook knowledge of gout but will talk as if they are an authority on it:

- I have woken up in the middle of the night with ripping, stabbing, throbbing pain in my toe or my ankle or my knee.

- I have had to take days off work due to the throbbing pain in my joints that won't allow me to put on a sock, let alone a shoe.

- I have had to sleep on the sofa because I can't make it upstairs because of the pain.

- I have had to buy a walking stick, and limp and hobble for weeks because of the pure excruciating pain.

- I have had to wince and gasp when my gout is suddenly moved or touched and the needles stab at my joints.

- I have had to give up all the normal food I eat and live on a diet of the most unappetizing 'healthy' foods.

- I have had to suffer through the physical pain and mental pleading and depression that come with every gout attack.

- I have had to learn what does and doesn't work for me and for others that I have spoken to.

- I have had to get to know my body and my condition.

- I have had to scour the internet and order books from libraries to get to understand the gout process and The Gout Danger Zone.

As a result, this book has been written not from the point of view of what makes doctors the most money, but from what will actually help you.

This book is written to make you aware of the process of gout within your body, and the causes of it from an ex-gout sufferer's point of view. It is the distillation of everything that I have learnt and experimented with over the last ten years,

It is an explanation of the problem of gout from a person who has gone through the cycle of:

HATRED OF THIS CONDITION

↓

FEAR

↓

UNDERSTANDING

↓

ACCEPTANCE

↓

RESPECT

↓

GOUT FREEDOM

So while there may not be a PhD or an M.D. after my name, there are over ten years of learning about gout first hand, from the trenches of the battle against this condition.

So, once again; simply put gout is an acid problem.

As your body processes the food and drink that you put into your body there are many complicated processes that have to take place.

All of these processes create waste products, just like when you make orange juice you end up with a lot of pulp, or when you drive your car the waste product is the fume vapour that comes out of the exhaust.

The same way when you eat and drink your body takes the nutrients to help it grow and stay strong from the food and also creates visible waste products:

Urine, Breath, Sweat and Faeces

We are taught to think of these things as bad, unclean and dirty, but that is not true. These are just things that your body doesn't need, want or can't process. Urine itself is sterile, sweat is almost 100% water, when we breathe out we breathe out vapour which contains many waste products that have been removed from the blood. Faeces, is well yeah that one's kind of dirty!

However, there are also waste products on a more chemical level too. As your body processes all the food and drinks you consume one of the chemical waste products/by-products of this processing is a substance known as uric acid.

The production of uric acid is normal for your body.

It is just part of how your body works, but when you suffer a gout attack your body has a surplus of this acid and it travels around your blood.

Think of this as similar to your household producing rubbish. On collection day you walk down the street and see every house with rubbish bins and bags out front waiting to be collected. This is what happens normally. Your body keeps on producing piles and piles of uric acid and your kidneys filter this uric acid to be removed through your urine.

However, in a gout attack there's too much waste produced at one time and your kidneys can not filter it all quickly enough.

Just imagine the rubbish your household makes over Christmas or Thanksgiving and then the collection men being on strike.

Your blood is loaded with uric acid during a gout attack and this causes the uric acid to build up and group together into crystals in your blood.

These crystals are shaped like microscopic javelins and they fly through your blood vessels as your blood is pumped through your body. They move easily usually until they reach a bend (a joint). Then they tend to get stuck, especially in the extremities of the feet and the hands.

This is the exact same thing that happens with water in a river; it flows fast until a bend and then deposits the silt and other debris it is carrying at the point the watercourse bends.

As more and more of these crystals get stuck in the joint they begin to kind of dam up the flow of blood. This doesn't stop the blood moving but does increase the pressure in the joint.

It is for this reason that the affected joint swells due to the increased pressure in the blood vessel.

This increased pressure pushes the sharp crystals into the soft tissue of your blood vessels causing pain.

The more crystals you have in your blood, the more severe the pain, the longer the attack and the less mobility you have in that joint.

Whilst the above explanation is not as scientific as a medical textbook would like, I hope it is graphic enough for you to understand the problem.

To summarize:

Basically in a gout attack you have too much garbage (acid) to be collected at one time and this garbage floats through your blood causing blockages in the joints.

Added to this is the fact that your muscles also have urate (uric acid) stored within them anyway. When under a gout attack, the condition of this build up of rubbish in your blood makes it easy for your muscles to push out the urate they store into the body creating a larger amount of garbage that needs clearing away.

This explanation is not meant to be scientific, but is meant to be for you the individual to graphically understand what is happening inside you when you suffer from gout.

"People wish their enemies dead, but I do not, I say give them gout, give them the stone!"

Mary Worley Montagu

Once again I remind you that I am not a doctor or medical professional but a real life gout sufferer and as a result the advice in this book is for you to follow if you wish.

2 TAKING PILLS

What I have learnt as I have suffered from gout over many years is that the simple idea of taking pills is a double-edged sword.

For me, sometimes pills will work and other times they won't. Sometimes pain killers will cause more pain than before I took them, other times they work perfectly. Sometimes gout tablets cure the condition other times they not only make it worse, but prolong it!

Talk about hit or miss!

Western medicine is very eager to treat every ailment and complaint with a drug, tablet or injection.

This can be expensive!

Western medicine is not a bad thing by itself as a doctor really is (or really should be) interested in getting you back to top health as quickly as possible.

However, with this said there is a problem with taking pills for gout.

Gout, or rather the appearance of gout in an attack is **not the problem**, it is the symptom of a problem.

The cause of the problem is not the gout, but all the other things that lead up to the gout attack and western medicine doesn't really address these causes adequately.

The doctor may vaguely explain changes we should make to our lifestyle and daily routine, but these are simply not good enough. This lack of clear explanation guarantees that you will suffer from further gout attacks in future.

Which nobody that has been through a full gout attack would ever want!

Gout mastery is about focusing and understanding the causes of gout. What is needed from you is a more hands on approach to the problem and a greater awareness of what is actually happening within your body leading up to a gout attack. This enables you to spot The Gout Danger Zone.

I am not advocating that you shouldn't take pills to cure your gout attack when it is upon you. That is not what this book is about.

If you find that the pills work for you, then take them.

If you find that they are not so good for you then don't take them.

Your medication is obviously your choice. What this book is all about is getting you the reader to understand that:

- To react to a gout attack is perhaps the worst way of living with and dealing with gout

- To live in fear of an attack is just as bad.

To be aware of the causes of gout attacks and the processes that happen in the body can enable you to see The Gout Danger Zone and get out of it before you even need pills or medical treatment.

3 ALCOHOL

Alcohol has a bad reputation when it comes to gout. Doctors are quick to advise the gout sufferer that alcohol is one of the causes of gout and that you shouldn't drink.

But then doctors advise everybody to stop drinking!

When it comes to gout, alcohol does play a role in the frequency and severity of the attacks you will experience. This is a simple fact, and any one that understands the condition and what is happening inside the body would never argue against it.

The traditional advice;:to steer clear of all alcohol is antiquated myth.

The relationship between alcohol and gout are not as clear cut as you may think.
This age old advice is also wrong and spoken out through ignorance:

`RED WINE AND PORT WILL GIVE YOU GOUT'

During a flare up when there is obvious pain, swelling and discomfort **you should avoid alcohol,** this I have tested and found to be an absolute truism!

Otherwise, when gout is not attacking you, when things are normal for you there is no real need to worry about alcohol so long as you spot The Gout Danger Zone and react appropriately.

So what is the deal with alcohol?

Through my years of trying to live with, and outwit gout, what I have found is that it is not the alcohol that causes the gout, it is not even really the quantity of alcohol that causes a gout attack, it is **the type of alcohol**.

I have found that wine whether red, white, pink, or fizzy, has no bearing on a gout attack. Through my years of experience and research I have learnt that wine itself does not induce or raise the risk of a gout attack. Old wives tales and old thinking may well disagree with this but wine is not the gout cause for me or perhaps even a trigger for gout.

Many gout sufferers I have spoken to would share this same sentiment:

Wine is Fine

BEER

All beer, whether lager, ale or stout is one of my true inducers of gout. There has been a lot of scientific research on alcohol and gout and as you investigate this it points to the fact that BEER IS THE ULTIMATE NO-NO for alcohol and gout attacks.

> **"…Beer consumption and, to a lesser extent, liquor consumption was shown to increase a person's risk for gout…"**
> http://arthritis-research.com/content/8/S1/S2

It is believed by many researchers that beer is the cause of gout due to the purine content. When purines are processed by your body the by-product is our old enemy uric acid once again.

Now since most people don't just drink one or even two beers, but more often have three or four, this becomes a problem. Having a beer or two after work is a habitual act for the majority of people, especially in Western industrial nations.

If you are in the habit of drinking beer often, it means that your body is kept in a **HIGH URIC ACID STATE** for a long period of time. As a result the chances of being in The Gout Danger Zone are high.

This means that your chances of going into uric acid overload (which basically means a gout attack) are permanently high too.

This is the problem for people that suffer from gout since this habit of having a beer after work, or a couple of cans while watching the TV does not allow your body to lower the uric acid levels in your blood to safer levels.

Therefore you are constantly very close to (if not in), The Gout Danger Zone.

This does not mean that a gout attack is permanently imminent, but it does mean that habitual beer drinkers may well have a hair trigger for attacks. Whilst this may sound a little dramatic, I have found that by: habitually drinking beer **INCONJUNCTION WITH** other risk factors does lead to a higher likelihood of a gout attack.

Now, all of this DOES NOT mean that beer has to be avoided. Not at all, but you must take care with beer to:

RESPECT THE DIFFICULTY THAT IT CAUSES YOUR BODY.

This does not mean that you cannot drink beer, but it means that YOU MUST HELP YOUR BODY to process beer and this is quite easy to do. Helping your body process uric acid more efficiently means that you must:

- Understand what you are putting in your body
- Think about the cumulative effect that this has on your system.

- Take preventative steps to minimize risk and maximize enjoyment.

SPIRITS

The other bringer of pain (both in the form of headaches and joint pain) is hard liquor. Whisky, brandy, vodka, gin, etc. if drunk with mixers are **not necessarily** a problem, depending on the strength of the drink you consume. However, if you enjoy drinking liquor neat, over ice or very strong then you are really placing yourself in The Gout Danger Zone.

Remember that your body processes all types of food, drinks and other substances with relative ease, but it is

THE QUANTITY THAT IS CONSUMED IN A LIMITED TIMEFRAME WHICH IS USUALLY THE PROBLEM

With hard liquor the amount of alcohol per shot means that a large quantity of uric acid is produced suddenly which needs to be processed rapidly by your kidneys. Ordinarily this is not a problem, but if you are in a **HIGH URIC ACID STATE** then your kidneys are already working hard and simply are unable to cope with the sudden influx of uric acid.

This places you in The Gout Danger Zone.

I have found through painful experience that if you drink shot after shot and don't take preventative steps then you are more than likely going to suffer for it by inducing a gout attack.

So, your job is to get to grips with your alcohol and assess it. I found that simply switching from beer to cider dramatically cut down my gout attacks from one attack every couple of months to less than one every two years!

To get your FREE Gout friendly food list

&

Gout Danger Zone check list, visit:

http://www.galexanderbooks.com/gout-free

4 DIET

One of the most difficult things for people that suddenly become gout sufferers is the fact that they have to change their diet.

Remember that gout is caused by your body breaking down the various foods and drinks which you put into your system.

This is very much like giving your body a mixed bag of good and bad ingredients and asking it to separate these out at the chemical level.

It is important with diet that you **do not** consider that you must avoid certain foods in order to remain gout free. This I have found is both a restrictive and joyless way to live.

By viewing some foods as good and others as bad we are not really allowing ourselves to control our diet, but simply relegating things which may or may not induce an attack.

You do not learn about your body or your condition this way.

When I first had a gout attack I went to the doctor and after the examination I was given a very simple explanation of how food affects my chances of having a gout attack.

The doctor basically explained that foods contain purines and that the higher the purine level the more uric acid is produced as your body processes it.

Whilst the explanation was both simplistic and old fashioned it was accompanied by a sheet of paper. The paper contained a list of foods to avoid at all times, foods that were very rarely to be eaten, foods which could be eaten often and foods that were okay all the time.

Indeed if you search forums online, most will offer similar advice and grim advice it is too.

The sheet of paper I was given was little short of heart breaking as all the good things that I liked to eat were outlawed.

Meat, poultry, shellfish and fish, eggs, beans, mushrooms and all other things that are requisite for any good recipe are gone.

Almost all online web articles do the same thing, telling you to cut out foods rather than educating you on what the foods actually do to your body. The great tasting foods are essentially replaced with, vegetables, more vegetables and fruit.

Meat, poultry, shellfish and fish, eggs, beans, mushrooms and all other tasty things are labelled as potential gout hazards and you are told to avoid them.

I ended up both depressed and at a loss as to what I could eat. You yourself may well have had a similar experience when you first learned you had gout.

The diet handed to me by the medical profession was to say the least; difficult to implement, soul destroying and boring.

However, as I have lived through my gout, I have learned that this list of hazardous items **OFFERS NO REAL EXPLANATION OR EDUCATION.**

By arbitrarily labelling a food as a gout risk you are not forced to understand your condition or how these foods can cause your body harm.

My body doesn't reject all these foods, it loves them.

Furthermore, this restrictive list as I look back now is some sort of fairy tale concocted out of ignorance rather than real research.

In fact, I was originally intending to call this book:

`Gout Free and Loving It in a Land of Beef and Beer'

The reason for the title was that I decided to test my understanding of gout, and The Gout Danger Zone by travelling through Vietnam for three months. Vietnam is a fantastic country with great people, weather, beaches, scenery, food, coffee and beer.

Beef, Offal, Shellfish and Red Meat

The most famous Vietnamese cuisine is a beef noodle soup called `pho', which is eaten for breakfast with strips of beef in every bowl.

This delicious soup is available in every city you could hope to visit and is simply the best thing to sort out a hangover (of which there were several). This meant that in the nearly three months of travelling **I ate beef almost every day.**

I know for some people (especially in western countries) the thought of noodle soup for breakfast is not that appetizing, but it's good ☺

Not only did I eat beef, but I ate all sorts of other taboo meats such as liver, kidney, intestines. I ate homemade blood sausage which was just intestines stuffed with mashed up offal and seasoning.

According to all doctors and websites supposedly giving advice I should have been constantly under attack from Gout. But I didn't have one attack, one twinge or difficult moment and had an absolutely fantastic time!

Due to the long coastline of Vietnam, seafood is another inseparable part of the cuisine, so I ate shrimp, crab and other taboo, purine rich foods like mussels and clams too. This was not occasionally, but almost daily.

Yet in all this time, I didn't suffer a single gout attack. Here I was eating beef for breakfast and having at least one other purine rich meal EVERYDAY FOR THREE MONTHS.

Not only did I not have an attack, I didn't receive even a twinge of gout in this three months.

The reason for this was the simple fact that **I understood The Gout Danger Zone.** I could spot when or if things were going bad and as a result I could take steps to get out of trouble before gout ever even showed up!

Did I mention that Vietnam has excellent beer?

Most people only know of Vietnam because of the war that the country suffered in the 20th century. Prior to that conflict the area was known as Indochina and was a colony of the French. France is famed for its wine and its beer and as a result Vietnam has excellent beer. This I enjoyed almost daily as my wife and I travelled around the country.

However I suffered no gout attacks and enjoyed the food and drink as if I had never suffered from or even heard of gout.

Is this to say that you should just eat whatever you like and you will remain attack free?

No.

The reason I could eat and drink what I liked was because of the simple understanding that I had about what gout truly is and how it affects the human body

By understanding and applying The Gout Danger Zone knowledge I had learned, I had the trip of a life time free of all the pain and problems. You too can do the same thing when you learn to spot The Gout Danger Zone. It is so simple once you understand what is truly happening inside your body, and remain vigilant to live a gout free life.

Processed Foods

Processed foods are everywhere in our diet, especially in the western world. This is not necessarily a bad thing on its own, but the amount of these foods that we eat can really have an impact on our chances of suffering from gout.

Just like drinking beer is not a problem, but habitual drinking is, so it goes for processed food.

Processed foods are filled with additives, flavour enhancers, artificial colours and other chemicals to prolong the lifespan of the food. All of these things are essentially chemicals. In other words they have been manmade or manipulated in order to make the processed food look more attractive to you so that you will eat them.

Your body is a truly marvelous piece of equipment, the amount of actions it carries out automatically would make even the smartest computer programmer blush. With this said, it is worth remembering that your body hasn't had an upgrade in terms of evolution for thousands of years. As a result these chemical additives and preservatives (which have only been invented recently) are not recognized easily by your body and many are difficult for your system to cope with effectively and dispose of.

A good way to understand this is to think how slowly a ten year old or even five year old computer works when presented with the most up to date software programmes.

Your computer might be able to run the programme but it will do so slowly and may well crash at times.

This is because your body just like the out dated computer will try and do the jobs it was designed to do rather than reject them.

Another major issue with processed foods is the fact that they contain a lot of salt. The reason for this is that salt is an extremely strong alkali and inhibits fungus and mould growth. Salty foods also taste good.

However, salty foods (processed foods) are quite hard on your body's system since they dehydrate the body and this means that you need to drink more water to counteract the dehydration.

Also the additives and artificial ingredients are quite toxic to your body since they are generally acidic in nature.

Fast Food

Fast food is basically processed food that is fried and as a result you get high salt, high artificial flavours, colours etc. along with, high fat content. These are in addition to the original nutrients of the ingredients which the body has to process too.

This is means your body will produce a high amount of uric acid following the burger meal or bucket of chicken

It is for this reason that fast food is an ultimate no-no when it comes to gout.

If you find yourself unable to give up the fried chicken or hamburgers, then don't worry or lose hope. These are not necessarily demon foods, but ones that should be eaten as treats rather than every day.

Once you learn to recognize The Gout Danger Zone and stick to the rules, you will find that fast food is something that can remain on your diet, (just not every day!).

With fast-food;

You must understand what it contains

How much it affects your uric acid levels

AND

Keep alert for the warning signals of The Gout Danger Zone

Time of Day

When you eat food your body has to digest this food and this sets into action various internal bodily functions. The whole digestive process is extremely complicated and pages upon pages could be written here about every chemical reaction and biological function. The majority of this science is thoroughly unnecessary for your understanding of what affects your gout.

The simple fact is that most gout attacks occur at night and this is due to two main factors; temperature and acid.

We deal with temperature in the `Heat' chapter, for now we'll focus on the acid factor.

Your body naturally becomes more acidic in the evening and this has to do with a whole multitude of things but mainly it is due to the food you have eaten, the fact that your body is getting ready for night time, and the change in the earth's magnetic field.

While this seems unrelated to diet, it can have significant consequences to your body.

If you eat a high purine, high acid producing meal late at night you are asking your body to process this at the worst possible time since it is at its slowest point and already more prone to being acidic.

It is therefore important with food that you get into the routine of eating several hours before you go to bed. This enables your system to process the food more fully and reduces the acidity.

Further to this if you can do some sort of evening activity such as walking or exercising this will move your body into a higher state of action and promote quicker digestion.

5 COOKING STYLE

What you eat is only part of the story when it comes to diet.

The other part is how the food is cooked.

This is SO IMPORTANT that it has its own chapter! SO don't shrug this off and ignore it ☺.

There is a great difference between fried chicken and chicken soup, not only in taste but also in gout risk.

This should be obvious to everyone.

When food is cooked the choices come down to three essential options:

Use heat (Barbeque, bake, grill etc.)

Use water and heat (steam, boil, poach, simmer)

Use fat and heat (shallow fry, deep fry, sauté, etc.)

Using heat alone or using water and heat to cook food are both excellent, healthy ways of cooking since they add no calories to the food.

Remember the food that you eat has to be processed by your body and so too does the way that the food is cooked. Therefore if you cook with water the body has to process water, which is easy for your body because it is 70%

water!

However, if the food is cooked using fat, this means that your body has to process not only the food itself such as beef or chicken, but also the fat that it is cooked in.

There is a great difference between bread and doughnuts, **even though they are essentially made from the same ingredients**, doughnuts are fried and bread is baked. One is cooked in fat, the other using just heat.

If you don't know how something at a restaurant is cooked there really is only one way to find out and that is:

ASK!

Sauces

Sauces play a large role in a lot of western food. We tend to have two types of sauces: water based or fat based.

Fat based sauces such as mayonnaise, tartar sauce, blue cheese sauce, Thousand Island dressing, ranch dressing etc. are greasy to taste. When we add these to our foods we are putting more fat on the food. This means our body has to process

- the food

- the way the food is cooked and

- the sauce we add to it.

Water based sauces are things like ketchup, relish, pickle, mustard etc. These do not feel greasy to taste. These are the healthier alternative to liven up your meal.

To find out if you are consuming a fat based sauce, then check if it tastes greasy.

Still not convinced?

If you put a little of the sauce on your finger and then try to wash it off with <u>cold water</u> the cold water makes the liquid fat in the sauce solid and as a result, your fingers are greasy / water sits on top of the shiny finger tip.

Another simple thing to do is look at the nutrition table on the label of the bottle.

The fat content alone will tell you. Mayonnaise is almost 90% fat while ketchup is less than 10%

The result of adding fat based sauces?

HIGHER URIC ACID PRODUCTION

This in turn puts more strain on your body and gets you one step closer to The Gout Danger Zone.

Simply opting for ketchup instead of mayonnaise can steer you further away from future gout problems.

To get your FREE Gout friendly food list

&

Gout Danger Zone check list, visit:

<u>http://www.galexanderbooks.com/gout-free</u>

6 FASTING

I myself have tried fasting in the past, with somewhat disastrous results. Yes I lasted for a few days without food and lost several kilos of body muscle and fat. But all that healthy fasting turned evil when it induced a gout attack and left me immobilized and in agony at home on the sofa, floor or in bed – whichever place I could get comfortable.

Fasting is likely to cause a gout attack for those that have previously suffered from gout attacks and for a very good reason.

When your body goes without food for a long amount of time (especially if you usually snack often or eat a lot) then to fill the food gap your body starts to breakdown your own muscle tissue and fat.

This is the reason that you lose weight when you fast, because your body has no food to process so it starts processing the surplus muscle and fat of the body.

This should be likened to eating a big piece of raw, bloody steak since the bodily process is the same.

Likewise if your body is in a highly uric state, that is to say that you eat a lot of meat, fats and processed food normally then it is easy to tip the balance and go into gout attack territory simply by skipping lunch and dinner in an attempt to lose weight.

The reason for this is because again uric acid is produced as a by-product as your body starts to breakdown excess body tissue.

Another issue with fasting is the fact that uric acid is actually stored in muscle tissues.

The reason for this is that although uric acid is the demon behind gout, it is beneficial for our bodies in the correct quantities. In the blood a constant supply is necessary to actually maintain healthy blood vessels; however too much uric acid just like everything else taxes the system.

Therefore when fasting the body processes muscle and fat and releases all this stored uric acid and if your body is in a high uric state then it overwhelms your system.

For a great book packed full of over 80 stress relieving techniques check out

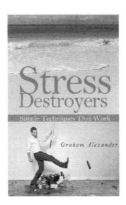

Stress Destroyers – Simple Techniques That Work

by Graham Alexander

Available at http://www.galexanderbooks.com/stress

7 HYDRATION

When it comes to gout, hydration basically means having enough water in your body. If you do not have enough water in your system this will move you into The Gout Danger Zone.

Doctors advise patients on the importance of hydration, especially during a gout attack, but the majority of doctors lack the understanding of how hydration works in your body. As a result the information doctors can give is limited.

People falsely assume that merely drinking more will make them more hydrated. However this is quite hit and miss since if you drink too much at one time your body doesn't have long enough to process the water before you have to urinate.

Trying to rehydrate yourself is often difficult because simply drinking water alone is not enough to guarantee hydration. Whilst this sounds a little crazy, it is true since the water that we drink whether from a tap or bought from a shop is most often acidic.

As a result our bodies expel most of this water through our urine without taking it in at the cellular level; therefore we do not fully rehydrate our cells even though we drink a lot of water.

Every bodily fluid is salty whether it is your tears, urine, sweat, blood, etc. What this means is that every time one of these processes is underway we are losing alkalinity.

This is the science behind sports drinks which, although these days come in many pretty colours, all share, (or should share) the same basic property and that is that they have an alkalizing effect on the body.

At the cellular level we need alkalizing fluids. These fluids enable the cells of our body to rehydrate. This is what speeds our recovery for sports and other things too.

In science class we learn that acid is one side of neutral and on the other side of neutral is the alkali or base.

These alkalizing fluids are marketed today as electrolytes, but in older times they were called salts as this is essentially what they are.

Salts or electrolytes are vital for the conduction of electricity from cell to cell within the body. A lack of alkalinity and cells don't function properly, a very simple example of this is muscle cramp through excess sweating.

Sweating too much too quickly causes sudden rapid loss of essential salts / electrolytes which alters the acidity / alkalinity of the body.

In the same way not drinking enough water causes slower but equally as dangerous dehydration.

However, most people, (doctors included) do not understand this basic fact and look to the macro level of drinking 2-3 litres of water a day and never fully understand the need for the alkalinity.

As we stated at the beginning of this book, gout is basically an acid problem and to combat an acid problem the use of an alkali / base is key.

One of the easiest ways to do this is to use bicarbonate of soda / baking soda as is discussed later in the book.

8 HEAT

Heat is one of the most controversial of all treatments for gout. The medical profession still advocates putting ice on the affected area to numb the pain and reduce the swelling whilst the pharmaceuticals do their work.

In forums and online chat rooms where **REAL GOUT SUFFERERS** say what works for them, ice is shunned and heat is recommended.

What is one to do?

For me personally I have found that heat works well even though my doctors all advised that ice should be used to numb the area.

At the beginning of this book it is stated that your body has limited ways to remove waste. These are urinating, breathing, defecating, and sweating.

Heat makes you sweat plain and simple. Even if this sweating is isolated to the skin of your feet, it is still the same process.

This may sound contradictory since we have just learnt about how we need to drink to replace our lost body fluids, but you must remember to replace them!

Your body strives to maintain a reliable temperature range of approximately 37 degrees Celsius. This is your core temperature and what this means is that the temperature surrounding your organs in your torso is kept at roughly this temperature. This temperature does fluctuate however due to times of day, year, diet etc.

As your body starts to heat up, your heart beats faster because it needs to send the hot blood away from your core to your limbs, fingers and toes in order to cool it down. As your blood travels away from your torso, it has more contact with your skin. The skin at your fingertips is cooler than at your core and this in turn cools the blood. One of the reasons that gout usually affects the toes is because they are as far away from your torso as possible and as a result the blood here is at its coldest.

As your body is heated whether through a shower, bath, sauna, heat pack, exercise or sunbathing it secrets water from the skin (sweat) in order to cool the blood through use of convection currents (the air on your skin).

This sweat is salty to taste since it is water from your body and is alkaline. However, sweat also contains a lot of the toxins that the body needs to get rid of and this is one of the reasons why saunas are good for your health.

The toxins removed from the body in your sweat mean that ultimately your kidneys do not have to process these in future. But this also means that

YOU MUST ENSURE YOU REPLACE THESE LOST FLUIDS
otherwise you will become dehydrated and closer to the Gout Danger
Zone.

However, heat is not only beneficial because of the toxins that are removed through sweat.

Heat works because it dilates the blood vessels which are under pressure due to the uric acid crystals that are built up in the joints blocking the flow of blood. When these blood vessels dilate the pressure is relieved, even if temporarily.

When heat is applied over a prolonged period of time the blood warms and this allows THE CRYSTALS TO BECOME MORE SOLUBLE AND ULTIMATELY MELT. It is the same basic science that is involved when you go to a coffee shop.

If you order a hot coffee they will give you a sachet of sugar crystals to add to your coffee should you wish. If you order an iced coffee you will be offered syrup, **NOT** crystallized sugar.

The reason?

Sugar crystals do not easily dissolve in the iced coffee, so liquid sugar is needed.

This is the same as gout crystals and cold blood. The crystals do not dissolve easily due to the low temperature.

So then, the aim is to heat the blood to dissolve the uric acid crystals whilst at the same time remaining hydrated and alkaline (since sweat also removes salts which keep the body alkaline).

There are many ways to help you do this:

Hot Showers and Baths

These are without a doubt the easiest ways to use heat for your own gout prevention. Take long hot showers or baths as often as possible. I have found that this is just great for gout, stress and general well being.

If you can't stand the heat then you should begin with a warm shower and slowly increase the temperature. As your body gets used to the warm water your heat tolerance level also increases. It is not <u>necessarily</u> the temperature of the water that is the problem when it comes to hot showers, but moreover the sudden change in temperature that causes us to be unable to withstand hot water. The more often you have hot showers, over time the greater your heat tolerance level will become.

Foot bath

This is my personal favourite, especially after a long day on my feet or when I just want to relax. I use a large plastic food storage container that is about ten inches deep. This I find is extremely useful as it bathes the foot and also my Achilles tendon quite nicely.

Saunas

These are great but may not be convenient since not everybody has access, but if you have a sauna at your local gym or spa, use it! Remember though to drink plenty of water or sports drink afterwards to rehydrate and re-alkalize your body.

Gout Socks

Cheap, effective and easiest to use, wearing socks in bed at night is great for keeping your toes and feet warm and this is important since, as we said at your extremities the blood is coolest. A thick pair of loose wool socks is my personal favourite.

Heat Packs / Hot Water Bottles

These should be used especially in the winter months, to keep feet warm. Another option is to use an electric blanket to ensure your body stays warm.

It is important that you realise the need to drink more water when using heat. If you come out of a hot shower, what this means is you have heated all of the skin of your body which means that the blood in your body has also been heated. Your natural response is to sweat to remove toxins and also cool the blood through convection currents. Therefore you must replace this fluid that you are losing.

Drinking several cups of tea or water will help.

Hot Drinks

It is very important that you understand the relationship of hot drinks and the body. In Oriental medicine, non alcoholic drinks are always to be consumed warm or hot, **NEVER ICED**. The reason for this is that your body needs to maintain a certain core temperature to function at its best.

Your body can sweat quite easily to cool itself down, or you can feel hot and remove a jumper or a jacket. However, when you are cooling your system down with iced drinks, it forces your body to expend a lot more energy trying to keep your core temperature warm.

From a gout point of view iced drinks are no good.

As was mentioned previously, if the blood is warm then the uric acid crystals dissolve more easily. Therefore you can assist your body's functions by supplying your body with hot (or at least warm) drinks which will act to heat you up from the inside.

One good way to do this is to have a flask of hot tea or coffee and have a cup every hour or so. Herbal teas are good for your digestive system too which will help with bowel movements and kidney and liver function.

If you like this book please help me by reviewing it on

www.amazon.com

or sharing it on face book. It would be a great help to me and also to all other gout sufferers out there!

The more reviews this book gets, the more people we can help!

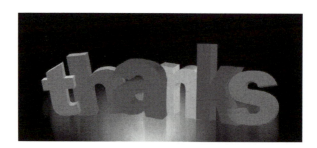

9 THE GOUT DANGER ZONE CHECKLIST

When it comes to gout, you should begin to view your body as a machine. The sooner you can adopt this attitude the better. Don't view your body as something that just happens, but as something that you can control.

Does this mean that you can control a gout attack?

Well, yes to a large extent you can.

A pilot has a check list of things that must be done before the successful take off of the plane and this is the same for you as you pilot your body through your life.

The Gout Danger Zone Checklist is:

Simple to use

but

MUST be reacted to.

If you drive your car and a red warning light comes on the dashboard, then you react to it. You do not ignore the light and hope the problem goes away. If you do sooner or later the car is going to breakdown and you are going to be stuck in a big mess.

This is exactly the same with gout. The warning signs that an attack is coming are there for you to see, but you must first:

Know the signs and react to them quickly.

Your body will give you all the time you need to alter your course so you don't crash head long into a gout attack. But you have to act quickly and without delay.

I have found through painful experience that if I ignore The Gout Danger Zone indicators, then a gout attack is sure to happen.

So what are The Gout Danger Zone indicators?

The difficult bit to get your head around is that The Gout Danger Zone indicators are more or less **PAINLESS.**

Once more:

The difficult bit to get your head around is that The Gout Danger Zone indicators are more or less **PAINLESS.**

The Gout Danger Zone indicators are slightly different for everybody, but all share a very similar core group of symptoms.

It must be understood that these symptoms are not the ones that you find on websites which explain the symptoms of gout.

Gout is the result of failing to notice The Gout Danger Zone.

While websites will tell you about the pain, stiffness and swelling in your joint, the heat and the agony, these symptoms are useless to you. If you already have these then gout is upon you and you are going to experience a lot of pain.

What the Gout Danger Zone does is allow you to stop the gout before it has a chance to develop into an attack. It allows you to notice what is happening and be proactive rather than reactive.

In other words instead of being a victim you put yourself firmly in charge of your body and your gout.

These warning signs may be different for you personally, so it is up to you to observe your body and take stock.

Apply this list to your body and heed the warning signs that you find.

The more you do this, the less surprising gout becomes. Instead, of suffering from gout, you begin to eliminate it from your life.

1) Check your feet.

If your gout attacks are usually in your hands or knees then check these areas instead.

Check your feet for any swelling. My first gout attack was in my left big toe, then following attacks moved to my Achilles and then ankle and then the outside of my foot.

However, through studying my gout attacks and keeping a close eye on my body, I have found that before there is any pain I have ample opportunity to stop the onslaught of an attack.

My left ankle will swell painlessly if I am approaching the gout zone. This swelling is usually around the ankle bone but then also include the flesh on top of the foot. If this looks puffy or inflamed or the veins are looking swollen then this is the red light on the dashboard.

Check your gout foot against your other foot to see if they look the same. I personally have never had a gout attack in both feet at the same time. Although it is possible it is very uncommon that both feet will be affected by gout at the same time.

If it is puffy this is a warning sign that your diet needs to change. This is especially true first thing in the morning since your feet have had the night off so all swelling from use should have gone down.

2) Check your urine.

For men this is quite easy. When you go to the toilet check your pee. What colour is it?

The darker it is the more dehydrated you are.

Whenever I get up in the morning I always check my urine. The reason for this is that during the night you breathe and sweat without knowing it and this removes fluids from your system.

Your urine when you wake up will be slightly darker than it should be, but it gives you a level to start from.

Also sniff your urine as you pee. This sounds a little strange but you can smell if your urine is salty or clear.

Drink water or warm tea or coffee as soon as you wake up, at least 250ml and continue drinking up to a litre over the next two hours.

When you urinate again check your urine to see if it has gotten lighter.

Keep checking it and monitor it constantly, this will tell you very quickly if you are heading into trouble or not.

I have found that carrying a bottle of water around with me is the best habit to get into. Yes I do end up going to the toilet more often, but at least this is pain free versus a few days of being incapacitated due to uric acid levels.

3) Think about what you have eaten.

This is perhaps the easiest tip since you can do it anywhere, whether driving home, in the office on the bus or watching TV. Assess your diet over the past three days. Think about what you ate and how you feel. If you have been eating a lot of fried food, meat or other so called `hazardous food' then think about what you ate and how it was cooked.

There is nothing more you can really do about it once you've eaten it, but by considering your diet, this should prepare you to be extra vigilant for warning signs of impending gout attack.

As a result you can now choose to have healthier options like fruit or vegetables. You can have a salad or a green smoothie, which taste great but look horrible! But are packed full of enzymes and alkali / base ingredients and will also make your digestive process quicker to remove the fast food from your system quicker.

4) How regular are you?

The majority of people that suffer a gout attack are also constipated at the same time. The key here is to check on yourself. Only you will know how regularly you sit down and squeeze one out and this is something that you should keep an eye on. Some people have one a day, other people have one every two days so I am not going to state that you should have one bowel movement a day because that is just wrong.

However, if you find that you have not had a bowel movement for longer than usual then this too is a warning sign that you should take steps to address. Simple ways to do this are to eat more vegetables and fruit or yoghurt. Other ways are to take pro-biotic tablets and powders. How you do it is up to you, but the simple fact is that you have to get the bad stuff out of your system. The swifter your bowel movements the less toxic your body becomes.

5) Stretch

This may well seem off topic but I have found it is very useful.

Anyone who has suffered from gout in their ankle or Achilles will know not only how painful it is, but also how rigid the muscles and tendons can become. This rigid, immovable state is caused by the uric acid that has been absorbed in to the soft tissue of your body over time forming as crystals. These crystals are medically known as tophi.

When you stretch your Achilles and ankle and knee joint what you are doing is assessing the flexibility of the tissue and the joint area and seeing whether or not the movement is hindered, slow or difficult. If you find that stretching is unusually difficult in one foot (your gout foot) then this too should be seen as a warning sign that the gout zone is not too far away.

10 THE EMERGENCY CUPBOARD

A long time ago a friend of mine taught me the following motto:

"Better to have and not need, than to need and not have."

Excellent advice for the gout sufferer!

Regardless of how competent you become at spotting The Gout Danger Zone and avoiding gout attacks, occasionally you will be surprised.

No system is fool proof and no one can remain vigilant all the time.

After all we're all busy people we have jobs to do, lives to live and kids to feed. Sometimes our best intentions get side tracked by the fast-paced life we live.

If you get to know and understand your body, you will be able to spot your own personal Gout Danger Zone signals before an attack occurs, but just in case you get caught out, you need to have an emergency cupboard ready for

QUICK SYSTEMATIC ACTION

Cherries

Cherries are hailed as one of the best and most reliable natural cures for gout. Cherry juice is well known to both help relieve symptoms and pain. I find it best to keep a couple of bottles of cherry concentrate in the cupboard or fridge. This is a very quick and easy go to when you feel an attack coming on and if unopened does not need to be refrigerated, so can be kept in the desk at work too or in the glove box of your car.

When cherries are in season I take advantage of any offers that may be on at the local supermarket and buy a lot and freeze them. They'll keep frozen pretty much forever and after 45 – 60 seconds in the microwave are ready to eat ☺

You can also take the time to make cherry juice ice cubes with concentrated juice. This is an easy way to add juice to a glass of water.

Green Powders

PH is important and to change your blood PH you need to be ready to deliver a lot of alkali quickly. One of the best ways to do this is through drinking rather than eating your vegetables and greens. Health food shops now carry wheatgrass and barley grass powders and both are packed full of alkali PH and are great for your body.

Avoid the darker spirulina powder as this is a high protein and therefore potentially high purine powder too.

I usually aim to drink at least one green shake, usually at breakfast time and then take another with me to work. They don't look too attractive but if made with the right ingredients then they are actually surprisingly delicious. (Especially if you use honey to sweeten them!)

You can drink these habitually as part of your gout combating regime if you like, but if not then keeping the powder in the cupboard just in case gives you a great weapon to fight uric acid.

Turmeric and Ginger

Turmeric is a natural anti-inflammatory amongst its many other properties and is effective in helping to relieve pain and swelling I have found. I combine a teaspoon of turmeric and a teaspoon of minced ginger (done in the food processor) and add boiling water to make about a pint altogether. I then drink this down like tea when it is cooled.

Honey can be added to sweeten as turmeric is quite bitter.

Ginger is also a natural thermogenic which means that it makes the cells in your body move faster and produce more heat.

Be prepared, for the very yellow colour of the turmeric!

Baking Soda (US) / Bicarbonate of Soda (UK)

This is without a doubt one of the most important parts of your gout emergency kit and should certainly be with you at work, at home and in your car. Bicarbonate is a natural alkali and has been used for centuries in medicine all over the world be it ancient Ayurveda from India, Western medicine or Chinese medicine, bicarbonate of soda / baking soda is a very powerful game changer for gout sufferers.

Whilst it is high in sodium, so should potentially be used sparingly (dependent upon your own personal health levels) half a teaspoon dissolved fully in a 200ml glass of water and drunk straight down four times a day reduces a gout attack from weeks long to days or even hours and it helps reduce the pain dramatically.

It is recommended that you drink a glass in the morning when you wake up and one just before you go to bed. The other two should be staggered evenly throughout the day.

One thing I do is have a one litre see through bottle (mine is glass, but plastic is fine) that I've marked on with a permanent pen the 200, 400, 600 and 800ml levels.

Then I take **two level teaspoons** of baking soda / bicarbonate of soda and put them in the bottle and fill with water in the morning.

I give this a good a shake and then this goes with me throughout the day.

Another successful thing I do is use the alarm function on my phone for my daily soda drinks.

This makes sure I don't forget to take it ☺

Medicines

For many gout sufferers medicines are controversial. Some sufferers swear by medication for gout, others can't stand the idea of them.

This is a judgment call that only you can make. If you want to use conventional medications, then it is a good idea to have at your disposal pain killers such as ibuprofen.

Gout specific medications such as colchicine and allopurinol are in most western countries only available on prescription.

However, with that said it is likely that if you have suffered an attack before you will have some left over medication.

I personally keep this in the refrigerator or freezer.

Most medicines lose their potency over time, but are also affected by excessive heat. It is therefore sensible to keep medications cool.

Whereas generally speaking I have found that colchicines and allopurinol actually make an attack worse in the short term, this is not the experience of everybody.

However, as with all conditions prevention is better than cure.

Therefore if you recognize you are in the gout danger zone, your toes or joints are becoming swollen, stiff or tingling with that gouty feeling, taking a tablet that you have used before and know the side effects of can see off the attack before it fully develops.

However, I stress here that this is your judgment call whether to take previously prescribed medicines or not.

Go Raw

Eating raw fruit and vegetables especially in a smoothie allows your body to take in massive amounts of nutrients, enzymes and fibre that all boost your immune system and digestive processes.

11 EFFECTIVE ACTION

"The best medicine I know for rheumatism is to thank the Lord that it ain't gout!"

Josh Billings

Gout is not a condition which can be ignored or forgotten about for long.

If you have had one gout attack sooner or later you are likely to suffer another.

To master gout it takes knowledge of your condition, which has been given to you in this book. But it takes more than that. We are taught to understand that: Knowledge is Power

But this is only half true. Knowledge is just knowledge.

<u>Knowledge plus action is power</u>

Gathering knowledge is like collecting money in a jar. It does nothing. It sits there on the shelf useless. It is only when you take that money and put it into action that you can buy things and enjoy the difference that this money brings.

In the same way with your gout, the knowledge of The Gout Danger Zone is useless unless you use it.

We have talked about the importance of understanding alcohol, diet, cooking style, hydration, heat etc. With this background knowledge you can now begin to implement it into your daily life.

The Gout Danger Zone has been explained to you and if you remain vigilant of your body and keep a check on what you eat, avoiding future flare ups is easy.

Do not be confused between the simplicity of the information you have been presented with and the ease of putting it into practice. You must work the key points:

1) **Check your feet.**
2) **Check your urine.**
3) **Think about what you have eaten.**
4) **How regular are you?**
5) **Stretch**

Check your body for any other personal warning signs too.

These points are simple, but so often overlooked. When you are feeling gout free and healthy you relax and become complacent. This is when you allow gout to gather together its forces and attack again.

By habitually watching for The Gout Danger Zone, you can steer your way to a future of fewer to no gout attacks.

It may take you another attack or even two before you start to accept your condition and begin to respect it.

The best way to think of gout is to imagine it as a sleeping dragon that only wakes up when you poke it too often and too hard.

Gout is totally controllable if you practice the key points and allow this to become a habitual check list.

To Your Bright and Boundless Future,

Graham Alexander

ABOUT THE AUTHOR

Graham Alexander suffered his first gout attack in his early twenties and suffered gout for many years until he began to master the condition. Through research, understanding and application of that which he had experienced, he developed his early warning system for gout.
He is from England and spent several years teaching in South Korea before returning to the UK. He is married and lives with his beautiful wife in the South of England

Other books by the author:

The language learning mindset book; *Free Your Tongue – What Your Language Teacher Won't Teach You*, a manual for anyone wishing to understand and control the mental hurdles to fluency in another language.

Teaching English in Korea – The Party's Over A serious look at the many reasons why the English teaching industry in Korea is going to suffer huge employment and pay problems over the coming years.

How To Quit Smoking For Life The author's own five step plan to quitting smoking without the use of gum, patches, vapour cigarettes or any other substitute. Based on scientific and psychological study, this book provides any smoker with the power to quit, through developing awareness and understanding.

Stress Destroyers – Simple Techniques That Work is a collection of highly effective techniques and methods to relieve and eliminate stress. Powerful tried and tested methods are combined in this excellent guide to reduce tension at work or home and develop more harmonious attitudes between partners, colleagues, friends and family.

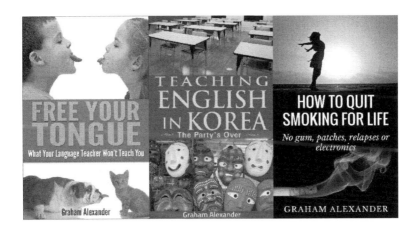

All books and other products are available at:

www.galexanderbooks.com

Printed in Great Britain
by Amazon